ON THE

TREATMENT, DIET, AND NURSING

OF

YELLOW FEVER.

(**FOR POPULAR USE.**)

By WM. H. HOLCOMBE, M.D.,
Of New Orleans.

BOERICKE & TAFEL:

NEW YORK, PHILADELPHIA,
SAN FRANCISCO, CHICAGO, etc.
NEW ORLEANS, LA., 130 Canal St.

TREATMENT OF YELLOW FEVER.

A PATIENT feeling badly should not "fight off" yellow fever and keep up as long as possible, but should go to bed at once, and begin the proper treatment.

Give him a warm foot-bath with a little mustard in it, and cover him with a sheet and two blankets. In very warm weather one blanket will be sufficient. Let the room be well ventilated, without any draught directly upon the patient. Hot orange-leaf tea is decidedly the best drink for a yellow fever patient, not to be forced upon him as a medicine, but as a means of quenching thirst, and at the same time keeping up a gentle perspiration. If that is distasteful or rejected, cold water (not ice cold) may be allowed, half a goblet about every half hour.

Purgatives are not necessary unless the bowels are very constipated, and then only the mildest should be employed. An enema of warm soapsuds is useful, and it should be repeated every day during the sickness, unless diarrhœa is present, when it will not be necessary.

There should never be more than two or three persons in the sick room at a time. Talking should be positively prohibited, and no conversation should be addressed to the patient. Do not worry him too much by trying to keep the cover close around him. There is no danger of his taking cold, and you may greatly injure his nervous system. Keep the room shaded but not darkened, and let no "neighbors" in any nearer than the front door. Never wake him from sleep for anything.

For the first two or three days, in the febrile stage, he needs very little, and yet a little nourishment. Offer him a little teacup of good black tea with a cracker or a small slice of toasted bread crumbed into it, about three times a day. If he wants nothing, let him alone.

The above directions are of extreme importance in assisting the action of remedies.

Begin your treatment with *Aconite*,

3d. Put 10 drops into half a glass of water, stir it very thoroughly, and give two teaspoonfuls every half hour, until the patient is in a good perspiration, after which it need be given only every hour.

In mild cases the fever will go gradually down, and no other remedy will be needed for the febrile stage. If, however, after 12 hours, the fever is still high and the pains severe, prepare *Belladonna*, 3d, and *Bryonia*, 3d, 10 drops of each in separate half glasses of water, and alternate every hour; one tablespoonful for an adult, two teaspoonfuls for a child. This should be kept up until the fever has decidedly abated or is gone.

The vomiting which occurs in the first or febrile stage is not a serious symptom. Give 5 drops of *Ipecac*, 3d, in a tablespoonful of water after every vomiting, and it will soon cease. A weak mustard plaster kept on a little while over the whole abdomen, will be very serviceable.

Sleeplessness and restlessness at night is sometimes a troublesome symptom. Put 10 drops of *Coffea*, 30th, into one-third of a glass of water, and give two teaspoonfuls every 5 or 10 minutes. If delirium is present, *Hyosciamus*, 3d, is better; use in the same way. A warm foot-bath and gentle friction of the back and limbs, with a little Sedative Water, are here beneficial.

Sometimes the fever does not go down, and the case passes happily into the second stage, but the temperature keeps up, and brain symptoms occur, and meningitis is threatened. Then give *Gelseminum*, 3d, 10 drops to half a glass of water, and two teaspoonfuls every half hour; sponge the body occasionally with tepid water and cologne or bay rum, and keep the bowels open by enemas.

If convulsions occur, or are threatened, prepare *Cuprum Aceticum*, 3d, in the same way, and alternate with the *Gelseminum*, 3d, every 15 minutes. Do not risk the motion of a general hot bath, but give a footbath and wrap the feet up in towels wrung out of hot water. If convulsions occur, you may check their violence with a moderate inhalation of *Chloroform*, the room being well ventilated.

Nine times in ten, however, the fever goes nearly or entirely off, and the patient thinks himself well, which, however, is far from being the case. You must now give him *Arsenicum*, 3d, and *Lachesis*, 6th, alternately every hour, prepared like the other remedies, and 2 teaspoonfuls at a dose. You must drop the tea and toast, and give him milk and *Lime Water*, half and half, one tablespoonful every hour, between the medicines, or if that does not suit the stomach, as much good beef tea. If the stomach becomes very irritable, let all food alone, and give milk and beef tea alternately by injection every 4 or 6 hours, two tablespoonfuls or more of each at a time. If the patient is very weak, two teaspoonfuls of brandy may be added to each injection.

The symptoms likely to give trouble in the second stage are vomiting, exhaustion, hæmorrhages, and suppression of urine. Each is so important, it must be mentioned separately. The *Arsenicum*, 3d, and *Lachesis*, 6th, have a tendency to prevent these occurrences, and the *Arsenicum* particularly should be kept up all along.

Vomiting.—Milk and lime water sometimes checks it in the beginning, particularly in small children, but it cannot be relied on long. If the matters vomited are *sour*, give a few grains of *Carbonate of Soda* in a little water after every vomiting.

Ipecac, as before, may be still useful. But *Argentum Nitricum*, 3x, is the best remedy for the vomiting of Yellow Fever, especially when signs of black vomit appear. Give 10 drops in a tablespoonful of water every time the patient vomits. If that fails after a fair trial, give *Sulpho-Carbolate of Soda*, 5 grs., in a little water, after every vomiting. Iced champagne, mint and brandy julep, by teaspoonfuls, are sometimes very useful. An enema, carrying off the wind in the bowels, sometimes relieves the vomiting at once.

Exhaustion.—This makes the patient feel dreadfully nervous and restless, so that he thinks he is sinking and dying. It frequently results from over-purging, over-sweating, and a starvation diet. *Champagne* is the sovereign remedy for a quick relief—a teaspoonful every few minutes. Give also injections of beef tea and brandy, until the stomach can bear the gradual introduction of food.

Hemorrhages.—Whenever any blood appears, from the stomach, or from the gums, or nose, or throat, or in the discharges, put 10 drops of *Crotalus*, 6, into half a glass of water, and alternate with the *Arsenicum*, leaving off the *Lachesis*. Rinse the mouth out frequently with *Tincture of Arnica* or *Extract of Witch Hazel*, ¼ of a teaspoonful to half a glass of water. *Plumb. Acet.*, 2x, *Gallic*

Acid, 1x, *Terebinthina*, 2x, and *Ergotine*, 2x, are all good remedies for hemorrhages. *Plumb.*, 2x, and *Ergotine*, 2x, from the stomach and bowels; *Gallic Acid*, from the gums and mouth; *Gallic Acid* and *Terebinthina*, from the kidneys; and *Ergotine*, from the uterus. One of these remedies may then be given intercurrently between the regular medicines—a little powder of one or two grains at a dose, dissolved in a little water.

Suppression of Urine.—This alarming symptom may last several days without being fatal; so do not despair. When the kidneys begin to flag in their action, give 10 or 15 drops of *Sweet Spirits* *of Nitre* in some water between the regular medicines, until the secretion seems restored. Encourage the patient to drink water. Rub the lower half of the spine freely with hot alcohol, and put a hot flaxseed poultice over the lower half of the abdomen.

If these measures fail, make strong watermelon-seed tea, and get the patient to drink as freely of it as possible. Be careful that it is really a suppression of urine, and not a *retention,* with inability to pass it. In retention, the bladder is full to the feeling, and pressure on it is disagreeable to the patient. An injection of ice water into the bowels will sometimes produce its expulsion. In refractory cases, it can be drawn off by the catheter, without difficulty or danger.

Suppression of urine, with brain symptoms, such as stupor and smothering delirium, is very dangerous. Here *Apis*, 2x, and *Opium*, 3x, alternated every half hour, to the exclusion of all other remedies, and in conjunction with the external applications above advised, may still rescue the patient from the jaws of death.

If the patient seems to get worse, and all the above means have failed, there is still hope in *Carbo. veg.*, 12—10 drops in half a glass of water, and a tablespoonful every half hour, increasing the interval between doses as improvement occurs. At the same time rub the whole body with *sweet oil,* heated as hot as can be borne, and repeat this inunction about every six hours.

In the latter stages of Yellow Fever, intermissions and remissions sometimes occur from the admixture, no doubt, of malarial influences. Then *Quinine* is very valuable. If it cannot be tolerated by the stomach, give it by injection, 5 grs. to 2 ounces of milk every four or six hours, until 20 grs. have been given; or, in very young children, by rubbing it into the skin with sweet oil or lard.

During convalescence, give *China,* 3x—10 drops in water three times a day for a week.

Be exceedingly careful about the diet of your patient in the second stage and during the convalescence from Yellow Fever. No solid food should be allowed, until all danger is passed, and a while after. He should take food in small quantities and often. I give you a bill of fare: Beef tea and chicken tea, from which the fat has been carefully skimmed; rice gruel, milk, buttermilk, weak egg-nog, milk punch at night, oyster soup (carefully), oranges to suck, beef steak and mutton chops to chew and spit out; aleree, porteree, and finally soft-boiled eggs, etc.

A Yellow Fever patient should not be allowed to get out of bed for any purpose. He should be kept in the horizontal position. He should not be moved from one bed to another. His clothing should not be changed unless it becomes offensive. It is then better to change it than to run the risk of sickening his stomach by its odor. Sponging with warm water, with soda and alcohol, brandy or bay rum in it, removes the odor, and is very refreshing. Do not let your convalescent read, or listen to long conversations, or sit up too soon. After severe cases he is a perfect wreck, and needs the utmost care, perfect rest and quiet, gentle stimulation and nourishment cautiously introduced.

In fine, do not overheat and oversweat your patient, do not overfeed or underfeed him. Have no company in the room, no talking, no evidences of haste, or anxiety, or excitement about him or around him. Protect his sleep from all disturbances. Satisfy his natural cravings for water, air, and light. Do not worry him with over-nursing, which is sometimes a terrible mistake. Make him *comfortable* in every respect. Let every nurse remember that if anything makes a sick man feel uncomfortable, it will soon make him worse.

There are many other remedies which might be required in different and intricate cases, but the above is a fair synopsis of the medication, diet, and nursing of yellow fever patients which, in the hands of the homœopathic physicians of the South, have reduced the mortality of that dreadful disease from its old high averages to an average of about 6 per cent.

Wm. H. Holcombe, M.D.

LIST OF MEDICINES.

Aconite, 3.
Apis mel., 2x trit.
Argent. nit., 3x.
Arsenic, 6.
Belladonna, 3.
Bryonia, 3.
Carbo. veg., 12.
China, 3x.
Coffea, 30.
Crotalus, 6.
Cuprum acet., 3.
Ergotine, 2x trit.
Gallic acid, 1x trit.
Gelsemium, 3.
Hyosciamus, 3.
Ipecac, 3,
Lachesis, 6.
Opium, 3x trit.
Plumb. acet., 2x trit.
Sulpho. Carbolate Soda, Pure.
Sweet Spirits Nitre, φ.
Terebinthina, 2x trit.
Tinct. Arnica, φ.
Extract of Witch Hazel.

The above Medicines may be obtained from the Homœopathic Pharmacy of

BOERICKE & TAFEL,
130 Canal Street,
NEW ORLEANS, LA.

www.ingramcontent.com/pod-product-compliance
Lightning Source LLC
LaVergne TN
LVHW020635110826
845149LV00004B/1211

* 9 7 8 1 4 1 8 1 9 1 3 3 7 *